DECLARATIVE

DECLARATIVE

33 Statements *that* Changed *my* Life

Jules Swales

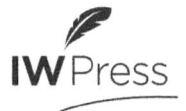

DECLARATIVE

First Published in Great Britain by IW Press Ltd
62-64 Market Street
Ashby-de-la-Zouch
England
LE65 1AN

https://www.iliffe-wood.co.uk/

Copyright © 2024 by Jules Swales

All rights reserved. No part of this book may be reproduced in any form or by any means without permission in writing from the author except for inclusion of brief quotations in a review.

Illustrations by Lara Czornyj
Cover design by 1981D
Interior design by Chapter One Book Design

A catalogue record of this book is available from the British Library.

ISBN-13: 978-1-8383330-9-6 (Paperback)

Introduction

Every human encounters challenges during their formative years. These challenges run the gamut and leave the young brain creating negative stories around the event and around themselves. Stories with "threat" or "lack" becoming woven into the human framework. Regardless of how "happy" a person's childhood, they still have a form of critical internal narrative.

These unconscious narratives dictate our future. They dictate how resilient we are in the face of rejection, loss, and betrayal; how we respond when someone cuts us off on the freeway, pushes in line in front of us, or simply disagrees with us.

The level of "threat" we experience depends on the level of our negative internal narrative. For some, the threat is done and dusted. For most people, the beliefs we accumulate from early lived challenges become the hazy lens through which we view ourselves and the world.

Every single person has a list of beliefs that hold them back from living their best life. *I'm not worthy, I'm flawed. I'm a failure. I'm insecure. I need to defend myself. I'm a bad person. I don't deserve to be happy.* To name but a few.

The important thing, the place of freedom, is for us first to recognize we have these limiting beliefs. Then to decide if we want to live our short precious lives, buried under their story.

Foreword

I am a writer and I have spent forty years studying humans. I'm fascinated by how we live and what impact early patterns of negative belief have on our choices, and reactions.

The following are a few traditional models used to combat negative beliefs: affirmations, cognitive reframing, identifying the belief, challenging the belief, or the "take the beliefs into therapy," approach. I've done them all and yes, they helped. However, none of them accessed the deeper, unconscious narratives, that were running my life.

One day I stumbled on a book *The Ultimate Coach*, written by Amy Hardison about her husband, Steve Hardison.

Steve has a process where he leads his clients to create their *Document*. Their *Document* is a list of personal statements, that originate from the *highest, noblest essence* of who you are. The essence he is talking about exists *at your inner core, the you without baggage, the you without wounds, damage, or fear.*

Did I have an inner core that was free of baggage? Did I have a high, noble essence?

And if so, could I find it?

Yes, I did. Yes, I did. And, yes I did.

This is my Document. I read it every morning and every night, and it has become the ethical principles from which I aim to live my life. Every statement is about me, and you can modify each one to be about you.

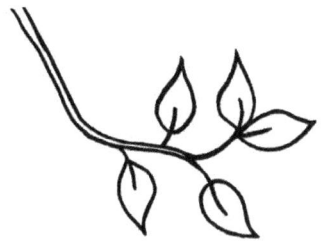

I am expansive, grounded, and high-reaching. The purity of a one true source. I am sheltered and resourced by this knowing.

Sensitivity is my superpower, tenderness, my tuning fork to truth. This is my offering to the world. I am gifted with an emotional internal landscape.

I lean into my sensory intelligence for guidance and direction. I am aware and aligned with my body's life force, my Sacral Inner Authority.

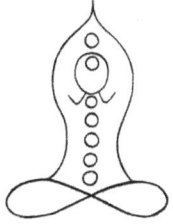

I live outside the boundaries of right and wrong in relationship with myself and with others.

I see the beauty of Soul
in every person I meet.

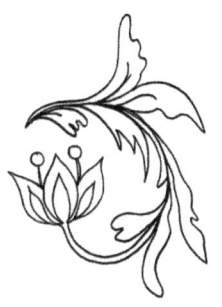

All my connections are rooted in compassion, kindness and respect. I am adored by those who know me. Friends, lovers, students, family, and strangers, all witness my uniqueness and my light.

My love has no container of word or deed,
it is my existence in the life of others that
is my gift of absolute love.

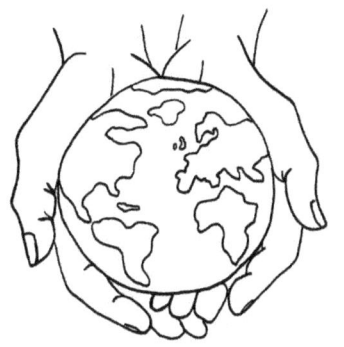

At all times I am divinely guided.

Every breath that I am is perfumed with imagination and power.

I am a generator of life force and have a magnetic aura that pulls towards me what I want.

I am patient and loyal to my business. I listen for her guidance and I respond. My business and my life provide bountiful income and personal delights.

I am a wise and generous teacher,
and leader.

I am grateful to have found my vocation. I adore what I do. I'm a profound and formidable receptor for those ready to work with me.

Words flow from me onto the page
and out to the world. My words are prolific
and entertaining as they educate and heal.

I am impeccable with accountability and self-efficacy.

Every moment of my life reflects my will and the will of the Universe in sublime reconciliation, balance, and harmony. The perfection of the Universe as cause, the perfection of me as result.

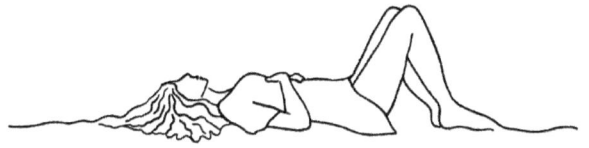

I am excited and enchanted to be alive.

I am free from ties, binds, or beliefs from the past, or past lives.

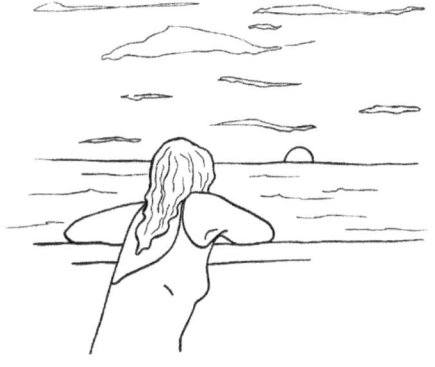

I have no reference or story of myself in former romantic relationships. Everything is new. I am ready and open.

There is a holiness and a dedication to the quality of my self-love, self-appreciation, self-focus, and self-care. I take time daily to check-in and honor my needs before all others. It is with intention that I cheerlead for myself. I am my priority.

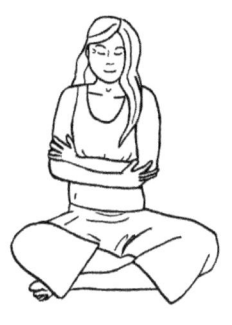

My body is my church, she is my jurisdiction. She is always beautiful and strong. I listen and trust my body. I care for her before all other things.

My life is alive with joy and happiness.

I am resourced by the deepest of knowing.
A faith that is undoubting and adaptable
in each unfolding moment.

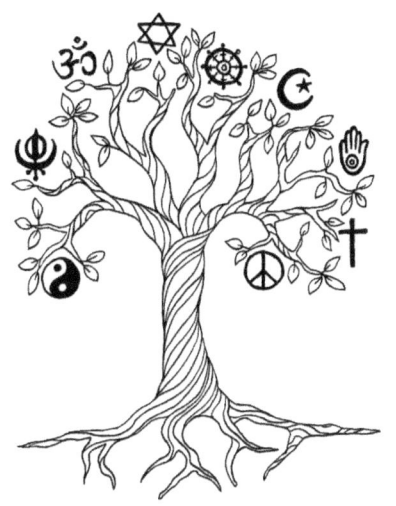

It is when I am most called to reflect outward that I first turn inward.

I have every strength, every answer, every understanding, and every freedom possible inside of me to comfort and support this journey.

My relationship with the Universe, with God, is sacred and steadfast. It is all love and all trust. And it is where I surrender and turn for guidance when I am worried or afraid.

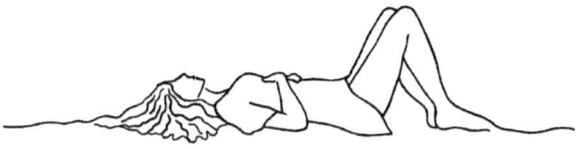

My relationship with myself is fiercely personal. It is patient, kind, and accepting.

My life is emboldened with curiosity and discovery.

In the majesty of a tree, a sunset, an early morning light, and the wind even, I am reminded that this same majesty breathes and lives as me.

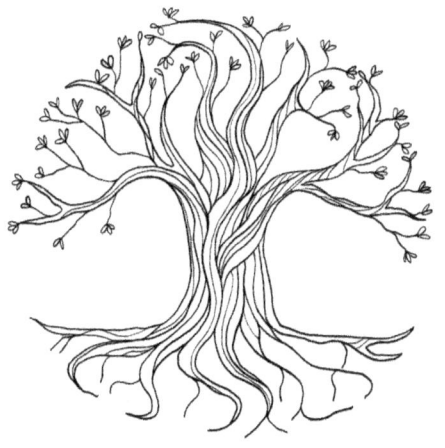

I am the current of a river, the force of the tidal, the puddles and rain. I am water, my life in eternal flow back to the unmeasurable vastness of ocean.

The Universe and I are sisters as body and soul.

And...

I am the precious gift to the world.

AFTERWORD

Words often have more to share with us than what we first write or what we first read. As an example here are the last eight statements of my document turned backward. This whole book of statements can be read backward, sentence by sentence. When I did that I was delighted at what more my Document had to share with me.

I am the precious gift to the world.
And...
The Universe and I are sisters as body and soul.
I am water, my life in eternal flow back to the unmeasurable vastness of ocean.
I am the current of a river, the force of the tidal, the puddles and rain.
In the majesty of a tree, a sunset, an early morning light, and the wind even, I am reminded that this same majesty breathes and lives as me.
My life is emboldened with curiosity and discovery.
My relationship with myself is fiercely personal. It is patient, kind, and accepting. And it is where I surrender and turn for guidance when I am worried or afraid.
It is all love and all trust.
My relationship with the Universe, with God, is sacred and steadfast.

About the Writer

Jules Swales is a published writer, poet and story-editor. She has a MA in Spiritual Psychology and a BA in Human Behavior/Interpersonal Dynamics. Jules runs an international writing school supporting writers around the world in connecting and perfecting their unique voice on the page. Her mission, through teaching writing, is to wake humans up to the splendor of who they are. She is known for saying: *We are not writing from our hearts; we are writing our way back to them.*

About the Illustrator

LARA CZORNYJ is a British freelance artist and illustrator. She studied art plus television and film set design. Her career began in art departments of the film and television industry. She creates in a variety of mediums, with her work often inspired by nature and her travels.

Resources

Many folks tackle the journey of creating their document on their own. Kudos to them. That approach wouldn't have worked for me. Too easy, too safe, nothing new. My Document would have been created from what was familiar to me, through my dirty lens. I needed a good window cleaner to point me somewhere fresh. That's where Sarah's program came in.

Sarah Steel – https://sarahsteelcoaching.com/

I have not worked with Steve directly, but I continue to read the book and want to give him a big shout out. I've always described myself as a spiritual scientist, I think Steve is a human scientist.

Steve Hardison – https://theultimatecoach.com/

www.ingramcontent.com/pod-product-compliance
Lightning Source LLC
Chambersburg PA
CBHW041309110526
44590CB00028B/4295